What **GOD** Wants You To Know About

Food & Health

One Rib Publications

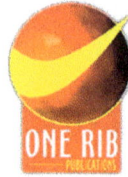

ONE RIB PUBLICATIONS
Nassau, The Bahamas
www.oneribpublications.com
oneribpublications@gmail.com

What **GOD** Wants You To Know About

Food & Health

Dr. Dave Burrows

Dedication

This book is dedicated to my friends, family, church family, and global family who seek a better and more fulfilling life. As always, my special thanks to my "wifey for life" Angela Burrows, and my children Arri and Davrielle. Above all, everything in my life is dedicated to God, for giving me life and sustaining me through the ups and downs.

Contents

DEDICATION v

INTRODUCTION viiii

CHAPTER 1
My Health Journey...1

CHAPTER 2
Understanding Food and Health: What God Said About It....11

CHAPTER 3
God's Health System 19

CHAPTER 4
Understanding Food..25

CHAPTER 5
The Journey to Excellence in Health......................................31

CHAPTER 6
Steps to Better Health 37

CHAPTER 7
Soul Health 45

CHAPTER 8
My Prescription Program for Better Health 51

SPECIAL NOTES 58

FINAL NOTES...62

HEALTH AND NATURAL REMEDY
INFORMATION AND LINKS...64

Introduction

The reason for this book is simple. Too many people are sick and are dying unnecessarily because they lack simple important information about food and health. Too many persons who call themselves believers are ignoring the words of God when it comes to food and health, thus negating their prayers.

This book is also a personal testimony about a journey to health that did not begin because of a textbook; rather, it was a real-life experience played out in real time affecting a real person and resulting in a health turnaround that is remarkable. This experience was indeed personal, and I am compelled to share with you this most incredible story that will leave you shocked, but also encouraged and hopeful, no matter what your current state of health may be.

Chapter 1

My Health Journey

Chapter 1

My Health Journey

Growing up, I never had health problems. I had bouts with the usual cold or flu, but nothing unusual. I was an athlete, playing baseball, basketball, running track, playing tennis, and swimming. I was somewhat of an ultra-athlete, running ten miles then playing basketball and wrapping it up with a swim of a mile. Through my teens and twenties I had no major health issues. In my late twenties and early thirties I began to experience fatigue intermittently; then it progressed to the point where the fatigue became constant. I also experienced joint pains and bouts of cold and flu. I had persistent mucus issues but shrugged these off because I had been healthy and active all my life.

These problems became acute during my thirties. I could not stand for more than a minute or two. I had headaches and extreme fatigue to the point where I took several minutes to make it upstairs one level in my house. Sometimes I would take fifteen minutes just to get out of bed in the morning. Not being able to explain my predicament, I began to see a number of doctors. Initially, they found nothing wrong. I had every test imaginable at some of the most highly regarded medical institutions in The Bahamas and the United States of America. Eventually, I was diagnosed as possibly having chronic fatigue syndrome (CFS) or Epstein-Barr virus. I was given medication, but the medication made me feel worse than I had ever felt in my life; so, I decided to discontinue it. At this point I decided also that I would just trust God and have faith to get better. I had been praying and believing, going through healing lines at church, having the "laying on of hands," meditating and fasting, but nothing changed. As time went on—a year or two—my condition worsened. My life became a nightmare. I was tired, aching, and at a loss as to what I could do to get better.

After mentioning my condition to several people, a friend heard about my situation and recommended that I see a chiropractor who also believed in nutrition and alternative treatments. I did not have much faith in chiropractors or alternative medicine; but, since I was still in a bad condition, I decided to visit him. The day I walked into his office changed the rest of my life and impacted my health forever. Certainly, it saved my life and prolonged my time on earth.

When I walked into the office, I was tempted to walk right back out, as the office was not impressive and caused me to wonder what he could do that the big medical institutions could not do. Finally, the doctor came out and asked me what my issue was. I started to state that I had been diagnosed with chronic fatigue syndrome. As I was finishing my sentence, he looked at me and said he knew that was not my problem. I asked how he could know it is not my problem, as my internal medicine doctor came to that conclusion after I had been examined at multiple highly rated medical facilities.

The chiropractor ignored my comments and went on to say that he could see what my problem was from looking into my eyes. Incredulous, I asked him to explain. He said that by looking at me, he could see that I was dehydrated and that I did not drink water. I quickly shot back that I don't drink water but I drink a lot of liquids, like apple juice. He explained that juice is not water and that my body needed water primarily; the lack of water would cause constipation and toxicity, because the toxins were not being flushed out of the body. He stated that my joint pains and headaches were all related to dehydration, and most of the other problems I was experiencing were related to toxicity due to a poor diet. He also explained that the medications I was taking for headaches and flu symptoms were adding to my condition by increasing the toxins in my body.

He asked me what I ate on a regular basis and explained how what I was eating was also magnifying my problems. I loved several foods from my childhood, and I had not relinquished them up to that point. I loved donuts, especially white powdered donuts and coconut glazed donuts. I loved fried chicken and fries, fried (cracked) conch, lobster, and shrimp, steak, and sodas. I did not like vegetables; and I did not eat fruits regularly. The chiropractor explained that what I described to him would cause my death if I continued. He asked me if I wanted to get better, and after I replied yes, he assured me that if I followed his plan, my symptoms would disappear in three weeks. I was not optimistic, because I had been sick for over ten years; but, wanting relief, I complied.

I commenced the plan immediately and began taking a natural fiber- based cleansing product along with a nutritional supplement that contained ground-up vegetables, grape seed, and other plant-based products. I began going to the bathroom on a regular basis for days on end, after not being regular for years. I started losing weight; the joint pains were diminishing; and I was feeling much better. My energy began to come back, and within a week most of the symptoms of chronic fatigue had disappeared. After three weeks I was much better than before and better than I had been in over ten years. I was excited and began changing my diet to consist of a mostly plant-based diet with lots of fruits and vegetables. I still ate meat at this time, but I had cut back a little on red meat.

4

I was on my way. Unfortunately, after I began feeling better, I reverted to some of my old habits, particularly eating sweets. I loved donuts, Pop-Tarts with the glazed coating, oatmeal cookies, and apple pie. After a few months of eating sweets and other "ole favorites," my health began to regress. One day after I had trouble breathing, I went to see the practitioner again. I asked him what he thought the problem might be; he laughed and said apple pie. We both laughed, and he told me that if I wanted to get better, I had to stick with the plan.

What transpired over the next few years was an up-and-down experience. I was a lot better than before, but I continued to have problems because I periodically longed for foods I used to love, and I would sometimes go on binges. I used to eat a box of Pop-Tarts in one sitting after a meal. I was better than before, but still experiencing some of the former issues. During these up-and-down years, doctors discovered a tumor on one of my kidneys. I had the tumor

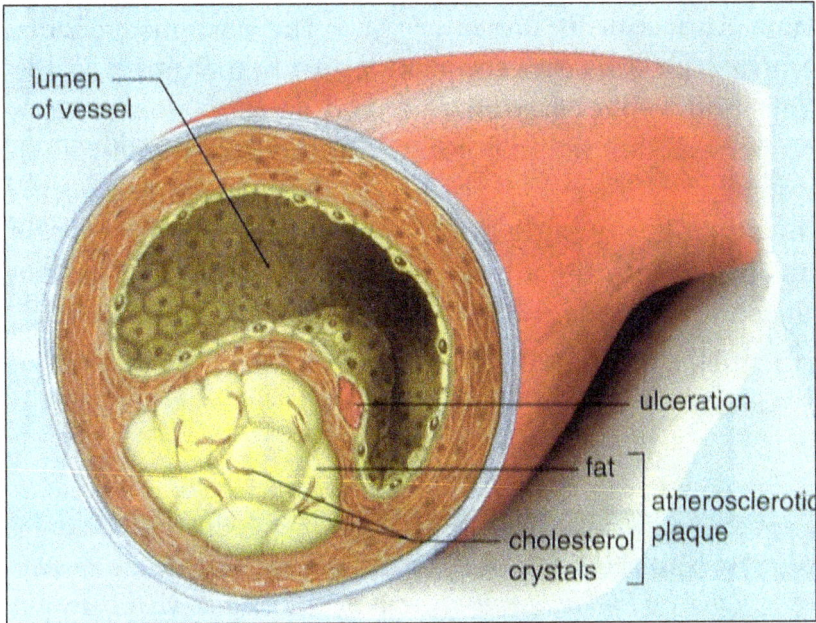

surgically removed in 2009 using a procedure called cryoablation. The doctor explained that cryoablation was a type of noninvasive surgery that required minimal hospitalization. The surgeon inserted a needle in the area where the tumor was and, through the substance in the needle, froze the tumor to death and removed it. The tests revealed that the tumor was benign but possibly pre-cancerous.

I recovered fully and was fine for several months after the surgery, until I went on a trip to London. At dinner my face became numb, and I wondered if I may be having heart issues or a stroke. I decided to go to the hospital. After a thorough examination, doctors could find nothing wrong and suggested I see a specialist when I returned home.

When I returned home I did not go to the doctor right away; but after experiencing indications of high blood pressure, I went. The doctor asked me to do a number of tests, including an extensive blood test, which revealed that I had high cholesterol and high levels of uric acid. The doctor then gave me a prescription for drugs to treat high cholesterol and another drug to treat uric acid. I let the doctor know that I only took medication as a last resort and asked if there was a way for me to correct the problem without the medication. The doctor indicated that to her knowledge this was the only course of action (although, she did mention that a change in diet might help). Being wary of medication, I decided not to take the medicines and instead decided to enroll in a natural health facility operated by medical doctors in Seale, Alabama, known as Uchee Pines Institute. My first day at Uchee Pines changed my life drastically.

I arrived in time for dinner. As I examined the food in the cafeteria, I noticed fruits, breads, and items—like chia seeds—that I did not consider normal food. So, I thought, *these foods must be the appetizers and the real food will show up soon*. I was told that what I saw was actually dinner. I was in shock. Right after "dinner" we were told to go to bed and in the morning we would see the doctor.

The next morning, I went to the doctor, who checked my vitals and took some blood samples. The following day, staff took more blood samples. While waiting for the blood results, we began classes, engaged in exercises, and received massages, hydro therapy, sauna, steam and hypobaric chamber treatments. Between treatments we went to classes, and I was again caught off guard.

The classes began by explaining to participants that most of what we ate was not food. As I asked questions, I learned that almost everything we ate that was white was not naturally white. So, the flour, sugar, rice, and other grains were bleached into whiteness. I learned that bleaching made no sense and actually destroyed the nutrients in the food rather than enhanced them. The instructors explained that after bleaching, vitamins and additives were added to put back things lost via bleaching (hence, "enriched flour," for example). They explained that the grains left alone simply as whole grains, unrefined, are much more beneficial. Processed, bleached foods, they explained, were totally unnecessary and only contributed to health issues, because the bleached food was not recognized by the body; the body was programmed to recognize things that came out of the ground, naturally. What a start!

The next few days I learned that what caused my high uric acid and cholesterol levels was the meat I was eating. And, I also found out that no meat was served at the facility. Not eating meat took some getting used to. When my blood results came back, they confirmed the diagnosis I had received at home: high uric acid and cholesterol. The doctors informed me that it would take only a week or two for me to see a reversal in my blood results.

At Uchee Pines we were forced to walk two times a day, breathing in and out according to a specific formula designed to increase oxygen intake (which was another issue I had—low oxygen levels). The instructors explained to me that most of the air I was breathing in was not air but recirculated air. They explained that I slept in air-conditioning, drove in air-conditioning, worked in air-conditioning, all of which meant that I was not getting adequate fresh air. It was beginning to make sense to me. And, I was also beginning to feel better. I began to embrace the process.

Next, I learned that dairy products were high in sodium and high in saturated fat and were the primary contributors to saturated fat intake, thereby creating many health challenges, particularly clogging of arteries resulting in blood pressure issues. They cut out my beloved cheese and milk. I was devastated because I loved pizza; but since I was feeling so much better—losing more weight, experiencing increased energy levels and alertness—, I decided I had to stick with the program, even if it meant giving up my most beloved foods, which led me to my next painful experience.

I learned that my body needed only a few milligrams of sugar per day and that one can of soda contained approximately 12 teaspoons of sugar. I learned that by the time I got to my apple pie and oatmeal cookies, my body was already extremely overloaded with sugar. They killed my donuts, cakes, and sodas. My beloved donut was a casualty of my new health program. I also learned that excessive sugar depletes and compromises the immune system, allowing viruses and bacteria to flourish. This was one of the reasons diabetics have difficulty healing from wounds—too much sugar was present.

Finally, they took away my beloved meat. I was informed that meat was the primary contributor to uric acid and one of the biggest contributors of saturated fats. So, my hamburgers bit the dust, my steak bit the dust, my lamb bit the dust; even my conch, lobster, fish…they all bit the dust. This experience was traumatic, to say the least, but I started to feel so good, I felt like screaming. I lost several pounds over the three-week period and my energy level increased exponentially. I learned that stress played a role in the process; so, I began working on techniques to lower stress. After three weeks it was time to re-take the blood tests. I sat in the doctor's office as, to my amazement, the new results showed that my uric acid level was normal, my oxygen levels were up and normal, and my cholesterol level had returned to normal. I needed no more convincing. I decided right then and there I would adopt the recommended vegan diet. That was eight years ago at the time of this writing. I have been (mostly) vegan ever since; and, although not free from health challenges, I have been much better. I have noticed that if I revert to old dietary habits, my problems resurface; so, for the most part, I stick to my diet.

I also learned to eat a big breakfast, smaller lunch, and no dinner at all or a very light meal at dinner. This way of eating was a completely new concept to me; but the nutritionists/dieticians explained that if you are going on a journey, you fill up at the beginning of the journey and not at the end. When you eat a big dinner, you are filling up at the end of your journey. I also learned that I should eat five hours apart, with no snacks between, because blood goes to where the food is, and digestion needs to be completed before introducing more food. I learned further that I should not drink with meals, because drinking prevents the secretion of enzymes in the mouth that are needed to break down the food for digestion. Therefore, I should drink water a half hour before a meal and one and a half hours after. I began practicing these habits and have adhered to them (with some slight deviations) to this day. I now drink water every day and in the appropriate amounts necessary.

Today I am healthier, happier, and living better because of the information I received; and this is the reason for this book. There were several persons who entered the same facility with me and were on as many as thirty-four medications a day; they left Uchee Pines on no medication at all. One person who was actually taking fifty-two medications and could hardly walk, left the facility a few weeks later walking miles at a time.

The benefits from my new diet and lifestyle included:

- No headaches, after years of chronic headaches
- Better skin
- No bad breath
- Increased energy
- No falling asleep after lunch at work
- No body odor, even without deodorant
- Weight loss
- Cholesterol reduction
- Uric acid reduction
- Mental alertness
- Increased oxygen
- No joint and muscle pains

My story is a firsthand account of health transformation through natural means. And I am here to help you get to optimum health through the same process I used. I know that for many of you this is too much to take in immediately. So, we have decided to approach it from three levels of transition that will be explained later in this book. You can do it! You may not be able to do it all right away like I did, but you can start. Do you want better health? Do you want to experience the results I received? Do you want to get off medication? Are you READY for the journey to better health? If you are, let's get it started.

Chapter 2

Understanding Food and Health: What God Said About It

Chapter 2

Understanding Food and Health: What God Said About It

Genesis 1:29
And God said, "See, I have given you every <u>herb that yields seed</u> which is on the face of all the earth, and <u>every tree whose fruit yields seed; to you it shall be for food.</u> (emphasis added)

Genesis 2:8–9 (KJV)
And the LORD God planted a garden eastward in Eden; and there he put the man whom he had formed. ⁹ And out of the ground made the LORD God to grow <u>every tree that is pleasant to the sight, and good for food;</u> the tree of life also in the midst of the garden, and the tree of knowledge of good and evil. (emphasis added)

Revelation 22:1–2 (NIV)
Then the angel showed me the river of the water of life, as clear as crystal, flowing from the throne of God and of the Lamb <u>down the middle of the main street of the city. On either side of the river stood a tree life,</u> producing <u>twelve kinds of fruit and yielding a fresh</u> crop for <u>each month. And the leaves of the tree are for the healing of the nations.</u> (emphasis added)

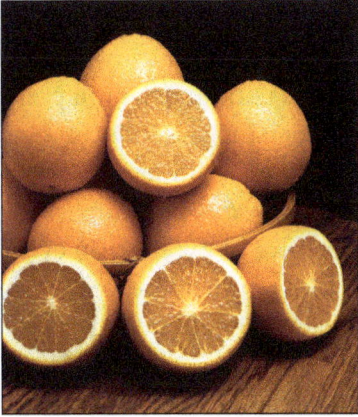

You will notice from these scriptures that the original design was for man to eat plants. Man's food was designed primarily to be herbs with seeds. This makes sense; because many scientists are now agreeing that man is not a natural carnivore. Man does not have fangs or a high-acid stomach to break down meats as efficiently as carnivores. Carnivores can break down meats easily because they have highly acidic stomachs. Man's body is more alkaline-based and is not ideally suited for meat as a primary dietary option, which is what we have adopted over time. In nature, many of our closest "relatives," including monkeys and gorillas, do not eat meat primarily.

Man has changed his original diet to include more meat, dairy, poultry, and processed foods that were not part of the original plan. We have also changed the meaning of food from whole grains to white flour, white rice, white sugar through a bleaching process similar to what is used to bleach clothes and in industrial cleaning. The bleaching process takes away the most important nutrients and leaves us with food the body does not easily recognize, because we came from the earth and our food is from the earth. When we alter, process, and modify food, sometimes we end up with food that is not programmed for our bodies. Man has genetically modified plants and animals (hybrids) and injected them with hormones to speed up growth and increase the yield of crops and the size of animals, to the point where the food is not good for us. Our food is now actually contributing to illness rather than health.

God wants us to be healthy. But, to achieve this health, we must cooperate with Him. We must adhere to His plan. God is an excellent God, and He created us to be people of excellence. We should be excellent in every aspect of our lives, not just one or two areas. We are three-part beings, and God wants us to be excellent in every part of our being. This sentiment is expressed in the scriptures, as evidenced by this quote from 3 John 1:2: "Beloved, I pray that you may prosper in all things and be in health, just as your soul prospers." We see here that God's desire is that we be excellent in every area of life. There are times when we focus on being excellent in other areas of our lives and neglect to be excellent in health.

God established a system with principles that govern every aspect of life, including health. His system is based upon universal principles that can never be altered, because they came from Him. An example of these principles is the principle of replenishing. Everything to sustain earth was placed in earth from the beginning; the earth is self-perpetuating. God does not send things from Heaven to the earth, from a physical standpoint, because everything to sustain life on earth is already here. He helps us by giving us the principle of activation.

Another principle that God established is the principle of seed and harvest. Plants have seeds, animals have seeds, humans have seeds; and what you sow is what you will reap. The principle of seed means that the earth was never designed to run out; seed perpetuates life.

The principle of sustenance is another important principle. You are sustained by your source, sustained by what you come out of. We come from the earth, or dirt; so, we are sustained by where we came from. We come from the earth; plants come from the earth; therefore, we eat dirt. We are "dirty" people who are sustained by dirt.

A fourth principle is the principle of intrinsic healing. Healing is built into our bodies. The human body is programmed to heal itself. Sometimes we have the mistaken notion that doctors heal people. The truth is that no doctor in the history of the world has ever healed even one person. Doctors simply assist the body in healing itself by identifying methods and substances that assist the body. If you cut yourself, the doctor stitches you up; but your body heals itself. If your body does not heal itself, the stitches are irrelevant. If your body does not respond to medication, you will remain sick or die. The intrinsic healing power of the body is the key.

In the same way that our bodies are sustained by earth, our spirits are sustained by God. Our bodies come from the earth, but our spirits do not come from the earth. God breathed life into us to sustain our spirits, while the earth sustains our bodies. Man's spirit is not from the dirt; therefore, the dirt cannot sustain it. We are sustained by God's spirit.

The loss of physical health is one of the greatest problems in the world today. If you pay attention to the news, you will see constantly commercials for pills and products to help us stay healthy or recover from sickness. We hear of numerous health plans, like "Obamacare" in the United States and national health insurance plans in other countries. The further we move away from the original food plan, the sicker we are becoming. This issue will never go away or even get better if we do not return to the original plan.

While we will always have health issues, the key to success in health is in understanding the keys that God gave us to healthy living. If we go back to His original plan, we would experience much greater success in health than with the plans we have put in place, which are painfully and obviously flawed and have led to disaster.

The truth is that God has given us instructions and answers that form the keys to our health, but we have found a way to eat our way into early and unnecessary death. We continue to dig our graves with our teeth. Is it a good idea to ignore what God says and then expect results He promised? I should think not.

Let's review from the Bible some of the other statements God has made about our bodies and health.

Psalm 139:13–18

For You formed my inward parts;
You covered me in my mother's womb.
[14] I will praise You, for I am fearfully and wonderfully made;[a]
Marvelous are Your works,
And *that* my soul knows very well.
[15] My frame was not hidden from You,
When I was made in secret,
And skillfully wrought in the lowest parts of the earth.
[16] Your eyes saw my substance, being yet unformed.
And in Your book they all were written,
The days fashioned for me,
When as *yet there* were none of them.
[17] How precious also are Your thoughts to me, O God!
How great is the sum of them!
[18] *If* I should count them, they would be more in number than the sand;
When I awake, I am still with You.

Psalm 104:14–15

He causes the grass to grow for the cattle,
And vegetation for the service of man,
That he may bring forth food from the earth,
[15] And wine *that* makes glad the heart of man,
Oil to make *his* face shine,
And bread *which* strengthens man's heart.

We are told that we are fearfully and wonderfully made, and we are marvelous. We are also reminded that vegetation is our primary food. Our body makes us legal on earth. But most people don't pay attention to their bodies until they are old or sick (especially church people). I believe it is time we take a close look at God's instructions regarding our body. He tells us what to eat and how to live, and He calls the body "His temple". We should listen carefully and observe what He has said in order to achieve our best and healthiest life.

Chapter 3

God's Health System

Chapter 3

God's Health System

God's system is very simple and easy to follow; but we have complicated it. His system is based on the principles outlined in the previous chapter. God's system begins with understanding our natural health sources. These sources have been termed the "six natural doctors," or six natural health systems. Let's take a quick look at these God-given health mechanisms.

1. **Air** — Oxygen. God has given us oxygen because we are sustained by air. The problem is that we actually avoid the air He has given us to breathe; and this negatively affects us. What do I mean? Most of us wake up in the morning in an air-conditioned environment; we drive in an air-conditioned car; we work in an air-conditioned office; we exercise in an air-conditioned gym; and, we return home to an air-conditioned house. What is the problem here? you may ask. We have not been breathing fresh, original air. We are breathing modified, conditioned, recirculated air; therefore, our oxygen levels are not where they should be. Air is free, but we do not take advantage of the free air; instead, we pay for air that has been modified and has less of what we really need. The body needs oxygen in order to perform functions such as:

- create energy
- digest food in the body
- clean toxins out of the body
- fuel the body's muscles
- metabolize fats and carbohydrates
- transport gases across cell membranes
- strengthen the body's immune system
- manufacture hormones and proteins
- remove viruses, parasites, and bacteria
- keep the heart.

2. **Diet** – God has given us natural original food, but we eat processed modified food that our bodies do not even recognize. Our bodies actually fight against some of the food we eat as if they were foreign objects. Our bodies readily recognize plants, leaves, fruits, vegetables, and grains because these are designed to sustain us. When we modify or add additives, preservatives and other unnatural substances to foods that are meant to heal us and sustain us, we cause them to become enemies of our bodies. God gave us fruits with natural sugar, but we add sugar to them, producing sugar overload. Instead of eating vegetables in their natural state, we cover them with butter or oil or sugar, thereby defeating the purpose of the plant. We also genetically modify foods and inject them with unnatural substances, thereby causing our food to harm us. Plants are available for us in their natural state to sustain us. If we go back to eating naturally, we could eliminate many diseases and illnesses.

3. **Sunshine** – We were designed to receive certain benefits by being exposed to the sun's rays. The sun is there to heal us, eliminate certain toxins, give our bodies vitamins, and provide healing properties through our skin. The sun is designed to kill bacteria and viruses and give us vitamin D and other nutrients. However, we avoid this natural doctor and do not receive the

God-given benefits. The sun is a vital healing and health tool that we do not use as we should. Too much exposure to sun can be dangerous but underexposure is equally dangerous.

4. **Water** – Our bodies consist of 85 percent water. In order for us to live, we must continually replenish it with water. Water is continually being used to provide nutrition to cells and to cleanse our system of toxins. It is used to replenish, cleanse, and deliver oxygen and nutrients. Water is also important to our blood as a main ingredient of blood cells.

5. **Exercise** – Whatever does not move will atrophy or eventually die. Our bodies are designed to receive life from circulation. Exercise stimulates and increases circulation; therefore, the more exercise we engage in, the more oxygen gets to our cells and the more alive every part of the body becomes. Lack of exercise means poor circulation, which means lower levels of oxygen and nutrients reaching our cells. Exercise stimulates life and releases endorphins, strengthening the immune system and brain. Science indicates that our bodies consist of 37 trillion cells, each needing to be "serviced". Our bodies have about 5.6 liters (6 quarts) of blood circulating through the body three times every minute to service these cells. Any part of the body that does not move regularly will begin to slowly die. We are designed to move to cause circulation to take place, thereby providing our cells with increased levels of water and nutrients.

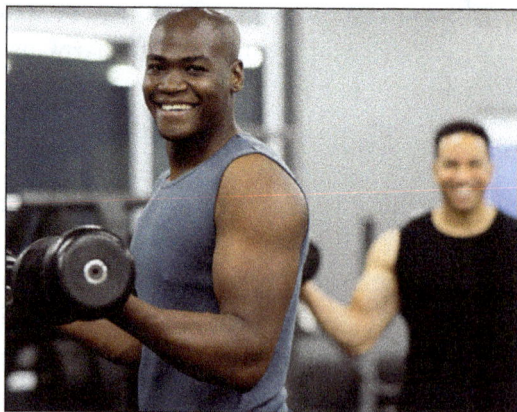

6. **Rest** – Our bodies are designed for activity and rest. The state of rest allows our bodies to recover from the stresses of activity and rejuvenate. The principle of rest was instituted by God when He rested on the sabbath day. When we do not get enough rest, our bodies do not recover properly, and our immune system is strained; so, rest is important.

These six natural doctors—air, diet, sunshine, water, exercise, rest—are there to ensure that we live healthy lives. If we neglect any one of these or any multiple of these, the result is diminishing health and future health challenges. Remember that these natural doctors cost you nothing but can save you from untold medical bills.

Once we understand God's system we must remember that when we go against God's health plan, we get sick and die prematurely. I learned this the hard way by eating excessive sugar and fatty greasy foods and not paying close attention to the six natural doctors. It is sad that it is only after we get sick that we panic and start to make changes which should have been made well before the onset of sickness. The journey to excellence in health is a very necessary journey, and it begins by understanding food: what is good food, bad food, God approved food. We must also understand how food has been changed by man for commercial purposes and determine what gives us the best chance for health.

Your body has a built-in immune system that fights viruses and diseases if it is properly serviced. The primary servicing of the immune system is through the six natural doctors. Everything in your body is designed to work by this system; even cuts heal because of this same system.

Chapter 4

Understanding Food

Chapter 4

Understanding Food

Man's original food was designed primarily to be herbs with seeds. This is borne out in God's original instructions in the book of Genesis.

Genesis 1:29
And God said, "See, I have given you every <u>herb that yields seed</u> which is on the face of all the earth, and <u>every tree whose fruit yields seed</u>; <u>to you it shall be for food.</u>

Genesis 2:8–9 (KJV)
And the LORD God planted a garden eastward in Eden; and there he put the man whom he had formed. ⁹ And out of the ground made the LORD God to grow <u>every tree that is pleasant to the sight, and good for food</u>; the tree of life also in the midst of the garden, and the tree of knowledge of good and evil. (emphasis added)

Man is not a natural carnivore. <u>Animals that are carnivores (primary food is meat) have high levels of hydrochloric acid</u> which allows them to break down meat so that it is easily absorbed into the digestive system. Man is capable of eating and digesting meat, but not as the primary staple of his diet. Most scientists suggest that man is more inclined to be an omnivore (capable of combination of plant food and meat). If we accept from the Scriptures what our primary food should be, and we recognize that we are not naturally equipped to consume large quantities of meat, it should become clear to us that our primary food should be plants. There is a tremendous debate raging globally as to whether the human diet should be vegan, vegetarian, or omnivore. I have personally chosen the path of veganism, simply because this is the path that has given me the best results for improving and sustaining my health. We will discuss the pros and cons further in this book; but for now, I will leave it to each of you to decide whether an omnivore, vegetarian, or vegan diet is best for you.

Man has changed his original diet and has changed what is considered food. It has been said that most of what we eat is not actual food that the body recognizes. We have bleached foods such as flour, rice, and sugar to make them white, and then further processed them so that our bodies, looking for the plants that God made, receive bleach and chemicals instead.

If that is not bad enough, man has genetically modified plants and animals and created a new class of foods called GMO or genetically modified organism. We are genetically modifying foods so that we can create crops that grow larger and faster for commercial purposes, without regard for how they will affect the human body. We have also genetically altered animals, injected them with hormones, antibiotics, and other substances that end up being transferred to the human population, producing "giants" and children who are anatomically advanced for their years, including females with breasts well before puberty. In addition, man has introduced many toxic pesticides and chemicals that not only damage the plants but seep into the soil, affecting our drinking water. The change in our food has had severe consequences, including the introduction and rapid multiplication of many diseases, including cancer, diabetes, high blood pressure.

The use of preservatives also impacts the quality of food, as many food preservatives have proven to be toxic. If we get back to God's original system, I believe we would get closer to His results. For us to achieve health, we must go back to God's original plan, His original food, and make it our preferred diet. How do we know this diet works? If we look at the Bible character Daniel, we would see that his story confirms the benefits of the original plant-based diet.

> Then the king instructed Ashpenaz, the master of his eunuchs, to bring some of the children of Israel and some of the king's descendants and some of the nobles, ⁴ young men in whom *there was* no blemish, but good-looking, gifted in all wisdom, possessing knowledge and quick to understand, who *had* ability to serve in the king's palace, and whom they might teach the language and literature of the Chaldeans. ⁵ And the king appointed for them a daily provision of the king's delicacies and of the wine which he drank, and three years of training for them, so that at the end of *that time* they might serve before the king. ⁶ Now from among those of the sons of Judah were Daniel, Hananiah, Mishael, and Azariah. ⁷ To them the chief of the eunuchs gave names: he gave Daniel *the name* Belteshazzar; to Hananiah, Shadrach; to Mishael, Meshach; and to Azariah, Abed-Nego.
>
> ⁸ But Daniel purposed in his heart that he would not defile himself with the portion of the king's delicacies, nor with the wine which he drank; therefore he requested of the chief of the eunuchs that he might not defile himself. ⁹ Now God had brought Daniel into the favor and goodwill of the chief of the eunuchs. ¹⁰ And the chief of the eunuchs said to Daniel, "I fear my lord the king, who has appointed your food and drink. For why should he see your faces looking worse than the young men who *are* your age? Then you would endanger my head before the king."

¹¹ So Daniel said to the steward whom the chief of the eunuchs had set over Daniel, Hananiah, Mishael, and Azariah, ¹² "Please test your servants for ten days, and let them give us vegetables to eat and water to drink. ¹³ Then let our appearance be examined before you, and the appearance of the young men who eat the portion of the king's delicacies; and as you see fit, so deal with your servants." ¹⁴ So he consented with them in this matter, and tested them ten days.

¹⁵ And at the end of ten days their features appeared better and fatter in flesh than all the young men who ate the portion of the king's delicacies. ¹⁶ Thus the steward took away their portion of delicacies and the wine that they were to drink, and gave them vegetables.

¹⁷ As for these four young men, God gave them knowledge and skill in all literature and wisdom; and Daniel had understanding in all visions and dreams.

¹⁸ Now at the end of the days, when the king had said that they should be brought in, the chief of the eunuchs brought them in before Nebuchadnezzar. ¹⁹ Then the king interviewed them, and among them all none was found like Daniel, Hananiah, Mishael, and Azariah; therefore they served before the king. ²⁰ And in all matters of wisdom *and* understanding about which the king examined them, he found them ten times better than all the magicians *and* astrologers who *were* in all his realm.

—Daniel 1:3-20

You will notice that this "scientific experiment" demonstrated that the original diet was superior to the man-orchestrated diet. I believe we should continue this test today, and we would see the same results, as I can attest to having personally undergone the same experiment.

Chapter 5

The Journey to Excellence in Health

Chapter 5

The Journey to Excellence in Health

God is excellent. In fact, He is referred to in the Bible as the Most Excellent. We are supposed to be people of excellence, just like He is excellent. The Bible tells us that Daniel was preferred because he had an excellent spirit. We can be excellent because God designed us to be excellent. Excellence in health is critical to every aspect of life. Excellent health keeps you here on earth. Excellent health makes you more alert, more relaxed, and more functional. I can attest to the tremendous benefits of excellent health. And I believe you will never regret good health.

God wants us to be healthy; but, as the Bible says, "My people perish —*literally*—because of a lack of knowledge." A lack of knowledge about your health causes unnecessary sickness and disease. The god of this world blinds the minds of unbelievers (2 Corinthians 4:4), and I believe we have been blinded and blind-

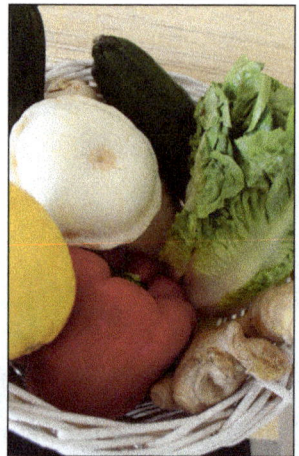

sided when it comes to health. I believe we all want to achieve better health; but exactly how do we do it? I know what you are thinking and what your question is: How do we achieve excellence in health?

It all begins with food.

Our bodies are programmed to receive certain components to function effectively, and when we do not receive those components, disease is created. Consider these statistics about eating the wrong foods.

- Nearly 75 percent of all deaths in the United States are attributed to just ten causes, with the top three of these (Heart Disease, Cancer, Respiratory Disease) accounting for over 50 percent of all deaths.
- New research estimates up to <u>440,000 Americans</u> are dying annually from preventable hospital errors. This puts medical errors as the fourth leading cause of death in the United States.
- Carcinogens and toxins (preservatives and additives in processed foods) in our diets are major contributors to diseases.
- Cancer that is caused by carcinogens and toxins results in unchecked cell growth. Mutations in genes can cause cancer by accelerating cell division rates or inhibiting normal controls on the system such as cell cycle arrest or programmed cell death. As a mass of cancerous cells grows, it can develop into a tumor. It all begins with toxins.
- Most of saturated fats come from animal products such as beef, lamb, pork, poultry with skin, butter, cream, cheese and other dairy products made from whole or 2 percent milk. All of these foods also contain dietary cholesterol.
- According to the American Heart Association:
- Polyunsaturated and monounsaturated fats are the two unsaturated fats. They are found mainly in fish such as salmon, trout, and herring; in avocados, olives, and walnuts; and in liquid

33

vegetable oils such as soybean, corn, safflower, canola, olive, and sunflower. Both polyunsaturated and monounsaturated fats may help improve blood cholesterol when used in place of saturated and trans fats.

- 65 percent of the world's population is lactose intolerant (unable to digest lactose in dairy products), with some groups as high as 90 percent.
- Trans fats (or trans-fatty acids) are created in an industrial process that adds hydrogen to liquid vegetable oils to make the oils more solid. Another name for trans fats is "partially hydrogenated oils". Trans fats are found in many fried foods and baked goods, such as pastries, pizza dough, pie crust, cookies and crackers.

Trans fats raise your bad (LDL) cholesterol level and lower your good (HDL) cholesterol level. These changes are associated with a higher risk of heart disease.

<u>Known toxins and carcinogens</u>
- Aluminum
- Alcoholic beverages
- Asbestos
- Tobacco
- Formaldehyde
- Salted fish
- Preservatives and additives
- High fructose corn syrup

<u>What our body needs vs What we feed it</u>
- Our body needs a maximum of 6 teaspoons of sugar per day; but one can of soda contains 14 teaspoons and one donut can contain another 7–10 teaspoons of sugar.
- Excessive sugar promotes tooth decay, slows healing, and promotes obesity.

- Our bodies need 2,300 mg of salt per day; but one slice of pizza can contain 1800 mg, and three slices of pizza would supply most or more than the recommended daily limit.
- Excessive salt is harmful to the kidneys and can cause any number of ailments, including kidney stones and increased blood pressure.
- Our bodies need unsaturated fats that come from plants such as avocado; instead, we feed our bodies cheese, which is highly salted and contains excessive levels of saturated fats. Meats, especially red meats, also contain high levels of saturated fats.
- Foods are designed to be consumed as close to the natural state as possible; instead, we fry our foods in grease containing high levels of saturated fats, which causes our arteries to become clogged, increasing blood pressure and causing heart disease, because the heart has to pump harder as the vessels narrow. This narrowing also makes it more difficult for the blood to circulate and supply nutrients throughout the body.
- Our bodies need plants, leaves, fruits, and vegetables; but we feed it chemicals, additives, preservatives, and other unnatural substances.

Doctors and Food and Nutrition

On the journey to better health, I must issue a caution as it relates to medical doctors. Doctors are there to help us, but we have to learn the truth about medicine and nutrients. Doctors are not capable of healing; we must realize that their job is to assist the body in healing itself. No doctor in the history of the world has healed a single person. They stitch us up and give us medication; but the body has to respond on its own. If the body does not respond, there is nothing the doctor can do.

Remember this: You should never have to go to the doctor for a problem you created. Medicine can save your life, but you are not supposed to live by medicine. Medicine is for intervention, especially lifesaving situations, but not as a lifestyle. <u>Medical doctors receive very little training in nutrition and health; their primary training is in medicine, which is not always the best route to health.</u> We should consult the six natural doctors every day before we have to consult a medical doctor. My recommendation is to go natural first (with caution), and when the natural is exhausted, go to the medical doctors. However, we should consult doctors for regular or preventive health checkups and tests to determine our levels of toxicity and indications of disease. Doctors are important for diagnosis of certain conditions and provision of urgent care. But reliance on medication can be deceptive, because in most cases the underlying health issues can be corrected by nutrition and lifestyle rather than medicine. There are some medications that are important in lifesaving situations; but as a rule, you should not pursue health by medication. You should produce health by natural food, exercise, and the other natural doctors.

Chapter 6

Steps to Better Health

Chapter 6

Steps to Better Health

STEP 1 – Eat Food The Body Recognizes

1. Go heavy on plants, grains, water, and foods closest to their natural state. Raw fruits and raw vegetables are excellent places to start.
2. Drink water above every other liquid, including juice.
3. When you cook, choose baked, boiled, or broiled over fried.
4. Most humans are lactose intolerant; therefore, do not consume any dairy products (cow milk, cheese, etc.)
5. Eat these foods: nuts (especially almonds), raw fresh vegetables (avoid canned and preserved vegetables that have high salt content) greens, brown rice, black rice, wild rice, spelt pasta, spelt flour, vegan or bean burgers, and vegan "meat," homemade vegetable soups with no cream (avoid canned soups or soups with high salt content and preservatives), vegetable pasta, whole grain bread, mushrooms.
6. Drink teas, because leaves are for healing. We should find which leaves are best for our health. For example:

   * White willow bark (for pain)
   * Echinacea (natural antibiotic)

- Golden Seal (immune system)
- Ginger or Lemon Ginger (digestion)
- Milk Thistle (internal organs)
- Dandelion root (internal organs)
- Hawthorn berries (heart)
- Saw Palmetto berries (prostate)
- Turmeric root (inflammation)
- Ginkgo leaves (memory)
- Cranberry (urinary system)

STEP 2 – Understand How To Eat

- Breakfast should be your largest meal, because you fill up at the beginning of a journey and not the end. Lunch should be smaller, and dinner should be very small and consumed before 6:00 p.m. The best recommendation is no dinner at all, only a healthy snack, because you do not need to fill up to go to sleep. When you fill up at the end of the day, your body stores the excess food, and your blood system works unnecessarily hard while you sleep. Remember: large breakfast; medium lunch; light dinner. "Eat like a king at breakfast, a queen at lunch, and a pauper at supper."
- Eat five hours apart to allow for proper digestion, with no snacks between your meals.
- Do not drink anything with meals, because liquids interfere with the excretion of digestive enzymes designed to break down your food for absorption. You will notice that saliva is produced when food is introduced into the mouth; saliva is what is supposed to interact with foods, not water and definitely not soda or fruit drinks.
- You may drink water 30 minutes before a meal and water or juice one and a half to two hours after a meal.

STEP 3 – Develop A Health Routine

- Develop a health routine that incorporates the six natural doctors.
- Begin each morning with a drink of warm water to stimulate your digestive system and to cause healthy bowel movements.
- Begin each day with meditation.
- Develop a habit of exercising regularly. Use aerobic (walking, running, moving) exercises first, as these are best for circulation and respiratory health.

STEP 4 – Identify Foods That Enhance Your Health

- Determine which foods are best for you and that your body responds well to. Remember: your body talks, and if you are wise you will listen. All of us are unique individuals, and sometimes our bodies would tell us that a food that is considered good for others is not good for us.
- It may be helpful to do an allergy test to determine if there are foods you are allergic to. I discovered after testing that the inflammation in my body was due to "nightshade vegetables," which may be good for others but not for me. Any foods with high acid content seem to bring negative results for me.
- Be careful even with natural products. The fact that a product is natural does not mean it is automatically good for you. You want natural foods, but you want the natural foods that are best for you.
- Learn proper herbs for your condition. Whenever you have health challenges, there are herbs that are helpful. Learn which herbs are right for you.
- Learn about conflicts and side effects. Many times we have seen advertisements on TV indicating the side effects of chemically

based drugs. Sometimes we also can experience side effects from natural products; so be vigilant about side effects even from natural products.

STEPS 5 – Identify Foods And Toxins That Harm Your Body

Check food labels for the following ingredients, and where you see them, avoid buying those foods.

- Hydrogenated anything
- Dextrose
- Preservatives (some of which are used to embalm the dead)
- Aluminum (Do not cook with it; it can get into your food and body system.)
- High fructose corn syrup. This ingredient has been scientifically proven to adversely affect health and is often used as a cheap sweetener. Use natural sweeteners instead; for example, honey, maple syrup, and Stevia.
- Trans fats and saturated fats. These are prolific in fried foods, fast foods, and many meat and dairy products.
- Aspartame, aspartate
- Cysteine, cysteic acid
- Avoid these food types:
- Pork (contains toxins, worms)
- Red meat (contains uric acid and is high in saturated fats)
- Scavenger animals and seafood (conch, shrimp, lobster) that collect waste from the earth or sea.

STEP 6 – Plan Your Perfect Healthy Day

What does the perfect healthy day look like?

1. Morning. The perfect healthy day begins early. Jesus arose early in the morning, before dawn, and meditated. What better example can we learn from. Your spiritual atmosphere is important; so, use your first hours to establish the tone of your day. The Bible tells us what Jesus did in the mornings: "Now in the morning, having risen a long while before daylight, He went out and departed to a solitary place; and there He prayed" (Mark 1:35). If God Himself prayed and meditated, then we should follow suit.

2. Praise and worship. Worship music sets the atmosphere and can lift your spirits.

3. Once you have meditated, exercise is important for circulation. It is always better to exercise outdoors, unless there is bad weather. Exercising outdoors allows for higher levels of oxygen intake. Walking and running are great, unless your joints may be negatively affected by running. Basketball, swimming, squash, racquetball, and many other sports are helpful for your conditioning.

4. Going to the gym is fine, but I favor outdoor activities. Air-conditioning is recirculated air and offers a lower level of oxygen. In addition to exercising, and especially as you get older, resistance bands can be very helpful. They provide great physical exercises and are easy to carry. I take my resistance bands to work or when I travel and use them at work throughout the day.

5. Of course, after exercising we should shower, shave, and cleanse our bodies of sweat and dirt. As much as possible, use natural products on your skin. I had a conversation with a dermatologist who told me that our skin ingests food; therefore, we should not feed it things that we would not ingest into our mouth. He recommended we use olive oil and coconut oil instead of chemicals, because the body recognizes natural pland-based oils.

6. Breakfast. I would recommend eating fruits along with whole grain cereals (hot or cold) or bread. I also drink tea each morn-

ing to get some leaves into my system. If you require milk, you should use almond milk, coconut milk, or rice milk. Do not add sugar to anything you eat in the morning. Use fruits as sweeteners. Hot cereals can also be helpful

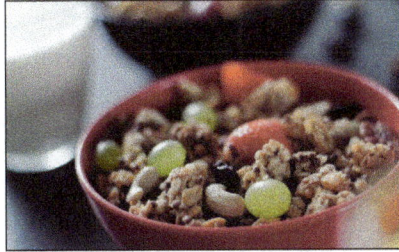

7. Once you have done the preceding, you should have a natural bowel movement, without strain or having to ingest chemicals. Using the bathroom regularly is a part of being healthy. If you are not using the bathroom regularly, something is wrong and needs to be addressed. In most cases, warm water, high fiber goods, hot cereals, and exercise should cure any constipation.

8. Lunch. Choose from these foods: nuts (especially almonds), vegetables, greens, brown rice, black rice, wild rice, spelt (or other whole grains like kamut or quinoa) pasta, spelt flour, vegan or bean burgers or vegan meat, vegetable soups with no cream, vegetable pasta, whole grain bread, mushrooms, chickpeas, and raw or baked foods.

9. Work. If you work in an environment where you are seated most of the day, get up often and walk around; do leg lifts while you are seated, which helps to firm up your stomach; and use resistance bands to keep your circulation up. Make sure you keep moving. Go outside, walk around the building, park as far away as possible when you are going to work or a shopping mall or event. The extra walk adds to your exercise regimen.

10. Take breaks. Go outside, take a walk and breathe deeply as you walk.

11. Make sure you drink room-temperature water at regular intervals.

12. Dinner. Eat light for dinner. I recommend bread, fruits, and nuts. Eat before 6:00 p.m. and do not eat again until morning. Dinner should be your lightest meal and should be consumed

before 6:00 p.m.

13. To end your day, do something relaxing to wind down and de-stress. Relax, study, meditate, and prepare for bed, ideally between 8:00 p.m. and 10:00 p.m.

Your routine may vary sometimes, but the principles above should not vary; these are the principles of a healthy day which leads to a healthy week and healthy year. Discipline is key, as stated in the Bible verse below:

> Do you not know that those who run in a race all run, but one receives the prize? Run in such a way that you may obtain *it*. [25] And everyone who competes for *the prize* is temperate in all things. Now they do *it* to obtain a perishable crown, but we *for* an imperishable *crown*. [26] Therefore I run thus: not with uncertainty. Thus I fight: not as *one who* beats the air. [27] But I discipline my body and bring *it* into subjection, lest, when I have preached to others, I myself should become disqualified.

—1 Corinthians 9:24–27

Chapter 7

Soul Health

Chapter 7

Soul Health

Physical health is essential, but health in your soul is even more important. Stress, worry, and anxiety have the capacity to negate your dietary changes and physical exercises and produce disease. Be very careful about stress in your life. Learn to take breaks, vacations, to laugh and find things you enjoy. Remember the biblical admonition below:

> Be anxious for nothing, but in everything by prayer and supplication, with thanksgiving, let your requests be made known to God; 7 and the peace of God, which surpasses all understanding, will guard your hearts and minds through Christ Jesus.
> 8 Finally, brethren, whatever things are true, whatever things are noble, whatever things are just, whatever things are pure, whatever things are lovely, whatever things are of good report, if there is any virtue and if there is anything praiseworthy—meditate on these things. 9 The things which you learned and received and heard and saw in me, these do, and the God of peace will be with you.

—Philippians 4:6–9

Remember that you are spirit first. Here is a scripture that shows us the preeminence of the spirit in our lives: "But the hour is coming, and now is, when the true worshipers will worship the Father in spirit and truth; for the Father is seeking such to worship Him. <u>God is Spirit</u>, and those who worship Him must <u>worship in spirit and truth</u>" (John 4:23–24; emphasis added). There is direct correlation between spiritual and physical health. Spirit affects body and mind: "He who begets a scoffer does so to his sorrow, / And the father of a fool has no joy. / A merry heart does good, like medicine, / <u>But a broken spirit dries the bones</u>" (Proverbs 17:21–22; emphasis added). This is why it is so important to maintain a healthy atmosphere and space in your life.

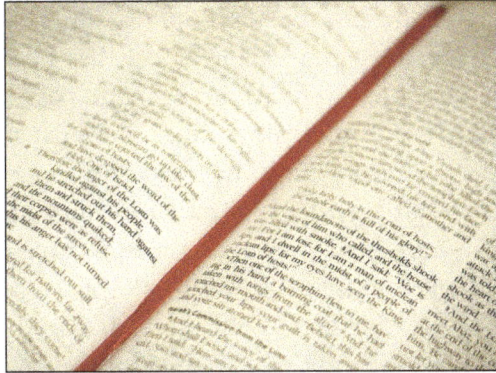

Consider this statement from a university study.

> Prayer is the most widespread alternative therapy in America today. Over 85 percent of people confronting a major illness pray, according to a University of Rochester study. That is far higher than taking herbs or pursuing other nontraditional healing modalities. And increasingly the evidence is that prayer works. It doesn't matter if you pray for yourself or for others, pray to heal an illness or for peace in the world, or simply sit in silence and quiet the mind—the effects appear to be the same. A wide variety of spiritual practices have been shown to help alleviate the stress levels, which are one of the major risk factors for disease. They also are powerful ways to maintain a positive outlook and successfully weath-

er the trials which come to all of us in life. The relationship between prayer and health has been the subject of scores of double-blind studies over the past four decades. Dr. Herbert Benson, a cardiovascular specialist at Harvard Medical School and a pioneer in the field of mind/body medicine, discovered what he calls "the relaxation response," which occurs during periods of prayer and meditation. At such times, the body's metabolism decreases, the heart rate slows, blood pressure goes down, and our breath becomes calmer and more regular. We call "this effect" the Holy Spirit.

Spiritual Prescriptions

This scripture is a prescription for a healthy soul.

> Rejoice in the Lord always. Again I will say, rejoice!
> [5] Let your gentleness be known to all men. The Lord is at hand.
> [6] <u>Be anxious for nothing, but in everything by prayer and supplication, with thanksgiving</u>, let your requests be made known to God; [7] and the peace of God, which surpasses all understanding, will guard your hearts and minds through Christ Jesus.
> [8] Finally, brethren, whatever things are true, whatever things *are* noble, whatever things *are* just, whatever things *are* pure, whatever things *are* lovely, whatever things *are* of good report, if *there is* any virtue and if *there is* anything praiseworthy—meditate on these things. [9] The things which you learned and received and heard and saw in me, these do, and the God of peace will be with you.

—Philippians 4:4–9 (emphasis added)

Remember that your physical and mental health are tied to your spiritual health:

My son, give attention to my words;
Incline your ear to my sayings.
²¹ Do not let them depart from your eyes;
Keep them in the midst of your heart;
²² For they *are* life to those who find them,
<u>And health to all their flesh.</u>
²³ Keep your heart with all diligence,
For out of it *spring* the issues of life.

—Proverbs 4:20–23 (emphasis added)

Remember that spirit affects mind, and mind affects body. Take care of spirit first. Everything in the physical, material world is a result of the unseen world. The unseen affects the seen. The unseen is eternal; the physical is temporary: "For bodily exercise profits a little, but godliness is profitable for all things, having promise of the life that now is and of that which is to come" (1 Timothy 4:8).

The physical has benefits, but the spiritual (eternal) is more beneficial. Do these things for better soul health:

- Pray
- Meditate on positive thoughts, participate in spiritually inspirational events and activities
- Relax (body and mind)
- Leave your normal environment (stressful environment)
- Fast (whole and partial)
- Enjoy nature (smell the roses)
- Be a peacemaker ("Blessed are the peacemakers…")
- Fellowship (socialize)
- Get massages
- Socialize with people who boost your spirit. Be around spiritually healthy people.

- Do not limit your thoughts, beliefs and perceptions of reality to the physical realm.
- Remember that God also provides supernatural, miracle healing.
- Believe for and expect miracles.
- But live by faith and not miracles.
- Think spirit first.
- Discipline your flesh. It needs to be disciplined and taken care of.
- Laugh. A broken spirit affects the mind, which then affects the body.

Chapter 8

My Prescription Program for Better Health

Chapter 8

My Prescription Program for Better Health

I realize that not everyone will move at the same pace and some people may choose to eat meats. Some persons may complete the journey in stages. Wherever you are on this journey and at whatever pace you proceed, the important thing to do is to <u>begin</u> the journey to better health. You can choose which steps are most appropriate for you and move at a pace you desire. But whatever you do, please get started on the journey to better health. Some of these steps are incorporated in previous chapters, so use this section as an overall guide through the process. Some of you may want to dive all in right away and become vegan, while others may take it more progressively. Therefore, I have created three levels of the program; you can choose at which level you would like to enter. I recommend you go directly to my level; but if you choose not to, at least begin with level one.

LEVEL I – Reducing Meat, Switching To Whole Grains, Reducing Salt, Sugar And Trans Fats

1. Switch to whole grains and natural foods. Use whole wheat flour, brown whole grain rice, spelt flour, raw sugar, and other whole grains instead of white flour, which is bleached. Look for "100%" whole grains (spelt, kamut, amaranth, millet, etc.).
2. Cut back or cut out meats. Meats have no fiber, cause production of uric acid, and increase calcium depletion causing osteoporosis.
3. Switch to raw foods as much as possible—nuts, greens, vegetables, and fruits.
4. Cut out grease (saturated fats). Saturated fats clog up arteries, causing high blood pressure and stroke.
5. Switch oils. Do not cook with extra virgin olive oil except at very low temperatures. Cook with coconut, avocado, or sunflower oils (look for high-heat versions).
6. Get rid of dairy. Use almond, coconut, or soy milks instead. Approximately 65 to 70 percent of humans are lactose intolerant. Cow milk is foreign to humans, is an allergen to many, contains unsaturated fats, and may cause the production of mucus (white blood cells attacking the foreign entity). As a dairy substitute you can also use cheese made from rice, nuts, or soybeans.
7. Use organic sweeteners such as maple syrup, Stevia (from the stevia plant), or honey (organic). Total sugar intake should be no more than 6 teaspoons per day. Fruits can also be used for sweeteners with cereal.
8. Eliminate peppers and spices except ginger, turmeric and garlic. Some spices and peppers are a major cause of inflammation and gastric ailments. Cayenne pepper may be an exception; but as a rule, use as little pepper as possible to prevent stomach irritation and inflammation in other parts of the body.
9. Bake, boil, or broil rather than fry, especially frying with saturated fats and oils.

10. Get sunlight and air. Indoor plants are good for eliminating carbon dioxide and providing oxygen, especially if you work indoors, with no windows. Get sunshine (at least thirty minutes per day) and breathe in four seconds, hold for seven seconds, and exhale for ten seconds. Sunshine is a great source of natural vitamin D. Remember: air-conditioning does not introduce new air but simply recirculates air. Lack of fresh air can lead to low oxygen, which is evidenced by yawning and sleepiness.

11. Exercise. Walk at least thirty minutes five days per week. Walking is best when done outdoors.

12. Cut back or cut out dinner, which should be the smallest meal. The largest meal should be breakfast and second largest should be lunch. Dinner should be fruit and bread, or light food.

13. Eliminate all sodas. Sodas contain up to 14 teaspoons of sugar and have no health benefit. Drink water (total of 64 ounces per day) and juice (sparingly). Do not drink "juice drinks"; they are just sugar and water. If you drink juice, make sure it is 100 percent juice. But remember that juices can be high in sugar also; so, consume sparingly.

14. Avoid medication, unless there is no alternative. Always research benefits and side effects. Many medications cause the need for other medications and do not provide a permanent cure. Medications can introduce a cycle of medication that multiplies.

15. Research natural treatments that have been proven effective. Get testimonials from people who have experienced genuine help. Look for verified research from double-blind studies in reputable journals. Check for verifiable results.

16. Do not drink with meals. You may drink water thirty minutes before meals and water or juice one and a half to two hours after meals. Drinking with meals interferes with the production of enzymes needed to break down food for digestion. When

food is "washed" down into your stomach, it has not been digested properly. Drinking with meals also causes stomach bloating ("beer belly").

17. Do not drink anything cold; room-temperature is best. Cold drinks may bind food to intestines.

18. Minimize sugar, especially refined sugars. Sugar depletes the immune system and inhibits its ability to fight bacteria and virus. Use natural sweeteners (fruits and fruit juices) instead of sugar.

19. Avoid synthetic foods (man-made or GMO-altered). Check for labels that state "non-GMO".

20. Eat right portions; do not overeat.

21. Eat five hours apart and do not snack between meals.

22. Drink water. The primary needs of the body are water, nutrients, and fiber. Drink a total of 64 ounces of water daily. Look for alkaline waters, such as Fiji, New Zealand, and Le Bleu.

23. Practice good digestion. Foods need saliva and enzymes to digest. Do not drink with meals, as fluids interfere with the production of enzymes.

24. Chew slowly to increase breakdown and absorption and to avoid indigestion.

25. Avoid acid-based foods. The body needs a pH above 7.0 for alkalinity. Get a pH tester and test your food and water whenever possible. Research foods that are alkaline-based and non-acidic.

26. Get an alkaline tester and an oxygen tester to test yourself.

27. Learn about the difference between medicine and health. You don't see a doctor until you are sick; doctors focus on prescribing medicine rather than on diet, exercise, and prevention.

28. Be very careful of hospitals. Hospitals are necessary and essential in some cases, but also are one of the leading causes of sickness and death. Ask questions about medications and research treatments to make sure you are getting what is best for you. Most hospitals are not very health or nutrition con-

scious. (Many serve sodas, GMO foods, foods with MSG, meals consisting of white flour, white rice, and the like. I visited a stroke patient in hospital and he was eating pork and drinking soda provided by the hospital.)

29. Be aware of harmful compounds and chemicals in hair products, household cleaners, cooking utensils (Teflon, aluminum, mercury, etc.). Teflon, for example, may peel from the frying pan and get into your food.
30. Avoid synthetic drugs (man-made chemicals). They should be used only after natural remedies have been exhausted.
31. Doctors are important, but understand their limitations. They have very little training in nutrition or preventive health; they are trained primarily in medicine. Find out if your doctor is up to date on food and nutrition.
32. Understand pharmacies and medicines. Pharmacies make a lot of their money from man-made products. You cannot patent or copyright natural ingredients; but most medicines begin with plants and end with the addition of chemical compounds that are synthetic and thus copyrighted and owned by pharmaceutical companies. These companies make more money the more medicine they sell, whether it is beneficial to you or not. Do your research on side effects.
33. Reduce salt intake (1-2 teaspoons a day maximum). Salt can have a negative effect on kidneys and increase blood pressure.
34. Avoid using the microwave; use a toaster oven instead.

LEVEL II – Adding To Level I By Allowing Only Fish, Chicken, Or Turkey Occasionally

1. All meat grass-fed or wild-caught. Mostly organic.
2. More raw foods.
3. No fried foods, only baked, boiled, or broiled.
4. Exercise at least four times per week. Use resistance bands.

LEVEL III – Full vegan diet, no meat or dairy.

1. Specific fruits and vegetables only (no hybrids).
2. Mostly raw food with only natural dressings (limes, sea salt, natural unprocessed sugars).
3. Cooked food that is primarily baked, boiled, or broiled.
4. Organic only preferred.
5. Follow the six natural doctors daily.
6. Exercise six days per week. Use resistance bands.

Special Notes

Check food labels carefully.

BAD INGREDIENTS
* Anything that says *Hydrogenated*
* Dextrose
* Preservatives (Some have the same ingredients used to embalm the dead.)
* Aluminum (Do not cook with it; aluminum can get into your food and body.)
* High fructose corn syrup
* Trans fats
* Aspartame, aspartate
* Cysteine, cysteic acid
* Monosodium glutamate (MSG). The following is a list of hidden sources of MSG:

    <u>Additives that ALWAYS contain MSG</u>
    o Hydrolyzed vegetable protein
    o Hydrolyzed protein
    o Hydrolyzed plant extract
    o Plant protein extract
    o Sodium caseinate
    o Yeast extract
    o Texturized protein
    o Autolyzed yeast
    o Hydrolyzed oat flour
    o Calcium caseinate

Additives that FREQUENTLY contain MSG
- o   Malt extract
- o   Bouillon
- o   Stock
- o   Natural flavoring seasonings
- o   Malt flavoring
- o   Broth flavoring
- o   Natural beef or chicken flavoring
- o   Spices

GOOD INGREDIENTS
- Organic fruits and vegetables
- Evaporated cane juice
- Organic maple syrup
- Whole grains (wheat, spelt, rye, etc.)

WHAT TO COOK WITH

- Coconut oil, sunflower oil, avocado oil (Check labels to determine if they are good in low heat or high heat.).
- Olive oil (only low heat, no frying).
- Be careful of salad dressings. Read ingredients and choose those that contain plants rather than animal fats or MSG or GMOs.

  - o   Remember the Six "free" natural "Doctors"
  - o   Sunshine – Natural source of vitamin D, which cures many ailments. Sunshine is good for fighting viruses and bacteria.
  - o   Fresh Air – Most air we breathe is recirculated, leading to lower levels of body oxygen. Oxygen is needed for all cells in the body; low oxygen level means low health.
  - o   Water – Our bodies are 85 percent water and we need water to cleanse our organs and systems of toxins. Lack of

water causes joint pains, headaches, etc., because toxins remain in the body. Drink eight glasses of water per day (64 ounces). Use high-alkaline water.

o Exercise – Without movement, circulation is limited, meaning there are parts of your body where blood is not flowing effectively. Low circulation results in deterioration.

o Rest – Our bodies need adequate rest to rejuvenate, which is why a sabbath day or day of rest was implemented. Lack of sleep or rest impacts the immune system, opening us up to disease.

o Diet – Plants, fruits, seeds are your most important food. The more raw plants and fruits you eat, the better. Drinking teas are also good, as they infuse your body with essential compounds.

Popular Foods and Alternatives

- Instead of hamburgers *use* veggie burgers
- Instead of cow milk *use* coconut milk or almond milk
- Instead of french fries *use* baked sweet potato wedges
- Instead of fried fish *eat* baked fish
- Instead of sugary cereals *use* organic grains
- Instead of white rice *use* wild rice, black rice, and brown rice
- Instead of soda *use* 100 percent natural juice
- Instead of white bread *use* whole grain, spelt bread

Vitamins and Supplements

Vitamins and supplements are fine, as long as they are natural-based and proper research is done to ensure that what you are taking is what is needed as a supplement to your health. Make sure that your vitamins do not cause side effects if combined with other supplements or medications. The most important thing to do is to research and consult with a nutritionist, preferably one who is aware of natural health and understands proper nutrition as has been outlined in this book. A vegan-based nutritionist would be helpful, especially if you have shifted to Level III of the nutritional prescription.

TEAS AND PLANTS FOR HEALTH

- Hawthorn berry (heart)
- Saw Palmetto berry (prostate)
- Turmeric root (inflammation)
- Ginkgo leaf (memory)
- Cranberry (urinary system)

Final Notes

CAUTIONS
- Make sure you get enough fiber.
- Use natural sauces and condiments that do not contain animal fats.
- Do not "dress" vegetables with butter, sugar, etc.
- Do not put fat or sugar on vegetables or fruits.
- Do your research on foods you eat and plan to eat.
- Consult with medical doctors who are aware of nutrition and favor natural cures.
- Consult with a professional trainer to determine what exercises are best for you and what regimen is best.
- Be careful with natural nuts. Over consumption of nuts can lead to kidney stones and complications because of excessive protein in your system.
- Get professional help, proper diagnosis, and tests.
- Healthy foods have effects: get educated about right foods for your issue.
- Try not to eat fruits and vegetables together.
- Get massages and use hot and cold therapy exercises.
- Look for home-remedy sites.
- We will help to provide information to assist in your journey from Level I to Level III. Please use contact information in this book.

Eating out?
What do I do when eating out? For many persons who have changed their diets, the challenge is how to combat the myriad bad food options at both fast-food chains and major restaurants. I have learned to creatively use the side dishes menus to create the healthiest options possible. For example: I go to a typical restaurant and

there is no obvious healthy option available. The first thing I do is ask if there is a vegan, vegetarian, or gluten-free menu available. If there is, I find suitable options from one or a combination of those menus. If no option is available, I create my own meal using healthy side dishes from the regular menu. In some restaurants, I would order avocado slices, sautéed mushrooms, sweet potatoes, brown rice, whole grain bread, vegetables, whole grain pasta or quinoa. If only white flour pasta is available, it is still healthier than other options on the menu when combined with the avocados, vegetables, and greens. Be creative, and you will find that you can create healthy options for yourself. You can also order salads with quinoa and nuts, or vegan burgers such as mushroom burgers or bean burgers.

Health and Natural Remedy Information and Links

Here are some of the health and natural remedy information and links that I have found to be helpful.

Understanding the global health and food problem
- http://www.worldatlas.com/articles/29-most-obese-countries-in-the-world.html
- *What the Health*, Netflix Documentary, 2017.
- http://www.pcrm.org/health/diets/vegdiets/health-concerns-about-dairy-products

Preparing and Eating the Right Foods
- Dr. Sebi's Cell Food, https://drsebiscellfood.com/
- Dr. Don Colbert, MD - www.drcolbert.com/
- Forks over Knives, https://www.forksoverknives.com/

Natural remedies
- GERD – http://www.ucheepines.org/gastroesophageal-reflux-treatment-protocol/
- Common cold – http://www.ucheepines.org/how-to-treat-a-cold/
- Dental care – http://www.ucheepines.org/dental-care/
- Sinusitis – http://www.ucheepines.org/sinusitis/
- Arthritis – https://www.ucheepines.org/arthritis/
- Indigestion – http://www.besthealthmag.ca/best-you/health/stomach-pain-relieve-gas-indigestion-and-belly-bloat-with-activated-charcoal/

www.ingramcontent.com/pod-product-compliance
Lightning Source LLC
Chambersburg PA
CBHW060256030426
42335CB00014B/1734